THE COMPLETE GUIDE ON THE SALAD DIET FOR BEGINNERS 2021/22

The definitive and updated recipe book on the Salad Diet, osing weight has never been so easy, build your diet daily thanks to the many recipes that I have created especially for you, an incredible variety of salads designed for beginners, easy and fast to prepare, but above all tasty, to the palate, the benefits will not take long to be felt.

Robert Sorrento

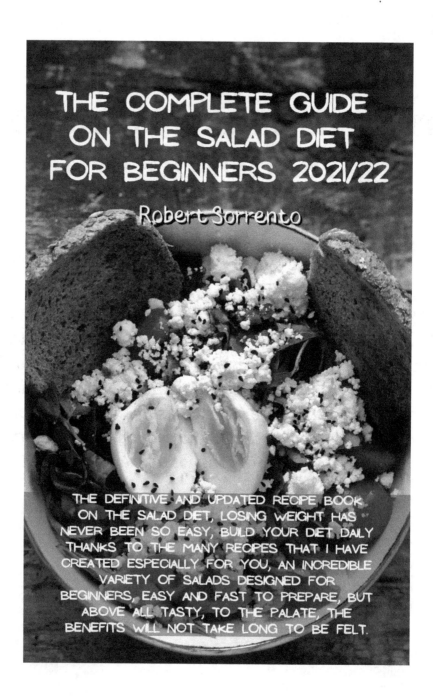

THE COMPLETE GUIDE ON THE SALAD DIET FOR BEGINNERS 2021/22

Robert Sorrento

THE DEFINITIVE AND UPDATED RECIPE BOOK ON THE SALAD DIET, LOSING WEIGHT HAS NEVER BEEN SO EASY, BUILD YOUR DIET DAILY THANKS TO THE MANY RECIPES THAT I HAVE CREATED ESPECIALLY FOR YOU, AN INCREDIBLE VARIETY OF SALADS DESIGNED FOR BEGINNERS, EASY AND FAST TO PREPARE, BUT ABOVE ALL TASTY, TO THE PALATE, THE BENEFITS WILL NOT TAKE LONG TO BE FELT.

Table of Contents

INTRODUCTION 10

GREEN SALAD 14

STEAKHOUSE WEDGE SALAD 15

WILTED SPINACH SALAD 18

WARM GOAT CHEESE SALAD 21

SOUTHERN CAESAR SALAD 24

CONFETTI CHIP SALAD 26

CLASSIC SPINACH SALAD 29

GRILLED ROMAINE 32

PASTA RICE AND COUSCOUS SALAD 34

LENTIL AND TRI-COLOR PEPPER SALAD 36

BROWN RICE, CORN, AND GRILLED VEGETABLE SALAD 40

CURRIED RICE AND CHICKPEA SALAD 43

GRILLED PORTOBELLO AND COUSCOUS SALAD 46

SUMMER BEAN SALAD 49

POULTRY MEAT AND SEAFOOD SALADS 52

....52

CHICKEN SALAD 53

MARGARITA CHICKEN SALAD 56

JALAPEÑO CHICKEN SALAD 59

FRIED CHICKEN SALAD 63

SOUTHERN FRIED CHICKEN SALAD 66

CHICKEN TOSTADA SALAD 69

CHICKEN FLORENTINE SALAD 72

TACO SALAD 75

THAI BEEF SALAD.. 78

GRILLED PORK TENDERLOIN SALAD 82

GRILLED LAMB AND TABBOULEH SALAD 86

FAJITA SALAD 90

SEARED SALMON OVER MIXED GREENS 94

TUNA NIÇOISE 97

SALMON AND ASPARAGUS SALAD 100

PANCETTA-WRAPPED SCALLOPS 104

SHRIMP STIR-FRY SALAD 107

LOBSTER SALAD.. 110

SPANISH SHRIMP, ORANGE, AND OLIVE SALAD........................... 113

MARYLAND CRAB CAKE SALAD... 116

VEGETABLES AND FRUITS SALAD 120

WARM POTATO SALAD 121

GREEK SALAD 124

LAYERED CHOP SALAD... 127

PANZANELLA 130

HEARTS OF PALM SALAD..133

GRILLED VEGETABLE SALAD 136

MANGO, AVOCADO, AND CILANTRO SALAD 139

ENGLISH FARMHOUSE SALAD 142

PEAR AND SPINACH SALAD 144

GRAPEFRUIT AND AVOCADO SALAD 147

WALDORF SALAD 150

FRESH FRUIT SALAD 153

WILDBERRY SALAD..156

TROPICAL FRUIT SALAD..158

CONCLUSIONS 160

The information in the following pages is broadly considered a truthful and accurate account of facts and as such, any inattention, use, or misuse of the information in question by the reader will render any resulting actions solely under their purview. There are no scenarios in which the publisher or the original author of this work can be in any fashion deemed liable for any hardship or damages that may befall them after undertaking information described herein.

Additionally, the information in the following pages is intended only for informational purposes and should thus be thought of as universal. As befitting its nature, it is presented without assurance regarding its prolonged validity or interim quality. Trademarks that are mentioned are done without written consent and can in no way be considered an endorsement from the trademark holder.

☆ *55% OFF for BookStore NOW at $ 31,95 instead of $ 42,95!* ☆

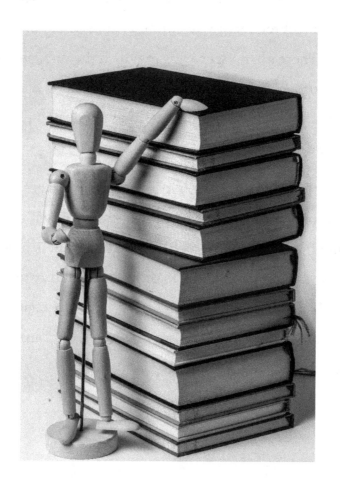

Buy is NOW and let your Customers get addicted to this amazing book!

INTRODUCTION

The salad diet is an excellent remedy to get rid of extra kilos and say goodbye to a swollen belly and heavy legs. Moreover, it is also a precious help to fight cellulite.

It is ideal not only in summer but in all periods of the year. Indicated especially after the Christmas holidays, it is very easy to follow. It is very popular among those who have little time to prepare lunch and those who, for work, are forced to eat out. If followed correctly, it is able to lose up to 5 kg in a week.

In order to enjoy its slimming effect, nutritionists suggest eating it at the beginning of a meal. This is a very popular habit among the French, definitely healthy because it hides several benefits for the body. First of all, eating it before lunch or dinner gives a sense of great satiety, which leads us not to overdo with the possible following courses, usually rich in carbohydrates and fats.

Here is what happens to those who eat lettuce
This also allows to shorten the time of digestion and effectively stimulate the metabolism. In this way, it helps to control blood sugar levels. In fact, the fiber

contained in the salad allows you to absorb less fat and carbohydrates in favor of the nutrients that are subsequently taken.

A salad diet allows for varying one's nutrition in a creative way. There are many types of salad that can be combined in a tasty way with vegetables and dried fruits. The most used varieties of salad are lettuce, escarole, iceberg, radicchio, and arugula.

In this cookbook, you will find a wide variety of salads revisited by me personally, and you will surely find recipes that will suit you both in terms of preparation and enjoyment.
All these different types allow, in equal measure, to fill up with nutrients and vitamins essential for the sustenance of our body. Here are the main benefits of salad:

- ✓ purifies the body: source of water and very little fat, it eliminates toxins and excess waste;
- ✓ it fights constipation: it brings precious fibers. Ideal for those who suffer from chronic constipation;
- ✓ antioxidant effect: especially green salads are rich in vitamins E and C, folic acid, lycopene, and beta carotene.

It is these nutrients that counteract cellular aging, as well as stimulate blood circulation;

- ✓ anti-tumor action: source of flavonoids, a valuable aid against the formation of cancer cells;
- ✓ defeats tiredness and stress: eating salad regularly allows to fill up with minerals such as potassium, magnesium, calcium-phosphorus as well as vitamin B6. The latter is useful, especially in periods of both physical and mental fatigue;
- ✓ help against migraine: lettuce, in particular, contains a substance called lactucarium that relieves headaches.

Start now this new path, build your daily diet thanks to the wide variety of salads that you will find here.

Robert Sorrento

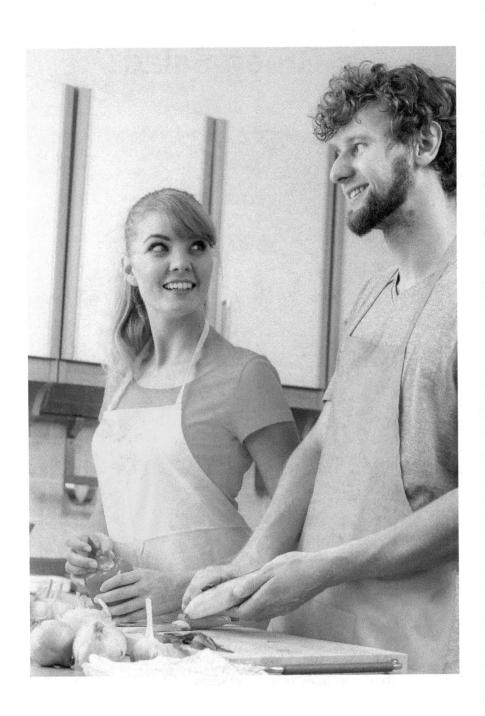

Green Salad

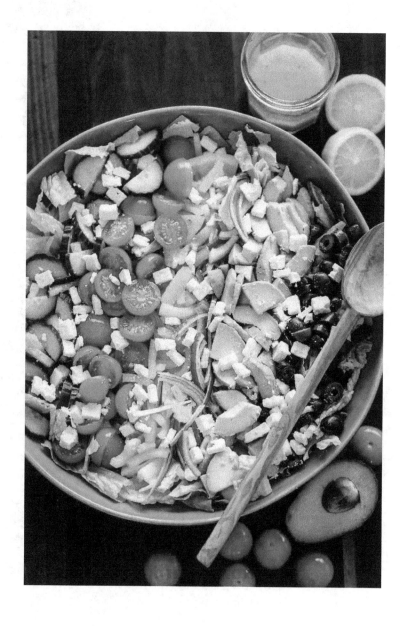

Steakhouse wedge salad

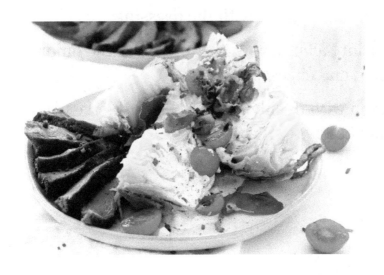

Serves 6

Ingredients:

1 bag (3 pack) Romaine Hearts

2 large tomatoes, diced

1 red onion, finely diced

½ pound bacon, cooked, drained, and crumbled

1¼ cups crumbled blue cheese

Freshly ground black pepper

Description:

Cut the romaine hearts in half lengthwise.

Place one wedge on each plate.

Generously drizzle with the dressing.

Pour into a large bowl the tomatoes, red onion, bacon, and cheese.

Season with freshly ground pepper. Serve immediately.

Wilted spinach salad

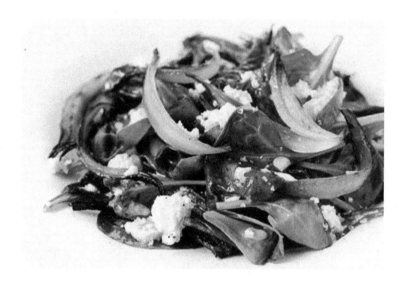

serves 4

ingredients:

One bag (6 ounces) Baby Spinach

¾ cup button mushrooms, cleaned, ends trimmed, and thinly sliced

Description:

In a large salad bowl, place the spinach and mushrooms.

Pour the hot dressing over the mushrooms and spinaches and toss gently.

Serve immediately.

dressing

Three tablespoons extra virgin olive oil

two tablespoons red wine vinegar

1 small garlic clove, minced

¼ teaspoon dried tarragon

½ teaspoon kosher salt

⅛ teaspoon freshly ground pepper

1 tablespoon sugar

1 egg, cracked into a bowl

In a small saucepan, pour the oil, vinegar, garlic, tarragon, salt, pepper, and sugar to a simmer.

Add the egg and whisk with a wire whisk until the egg is opaque and stringy and cooked through all the way.

Warm goat cheese salad

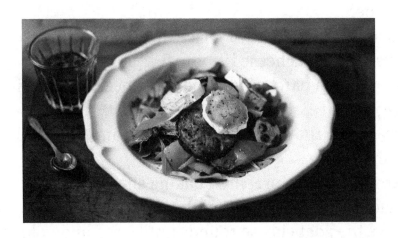

serves 6
ingredients:

salad
1 tablespoon olive oil
1 large egg
Kosher salt and freshly ground pepper
1½ cups plain bread crumbs
1 log fresh goat cheese, chilled in the refrigerator
1 bag European Blend

Description:

Position an oven rack to the highest setting.

Preheat the oven to 395°F.

Brush a baking sheet with the oil; set aside.

In a small bowl, whisk the egg with a pinch of salt and pepper.

In another small bowl, place the bread crumbs.

Slice the goat cheese log into 8 equal pieces.

Working in batches, dip the goat cheese rounds in the egg mixture, shaking off the excess.

Press into the breadcrumb mixture and pat gently to evenly coat.

Arrange on the prepared baking sheet.

Place the baking sheet on the top rack of the oven and bake the goat cheese rounds until crisp and golden, about 5 minutes.

Place the European Blend in a large salad bowl.

Add the vinaigrette to taste and gently toss.

Divide the salad among individual plates.

Top each salad with 2 warm goat cheese rounds.

Serve immediately.

grainy mustard vinaigrette

2 tablespoons white wine vinegar
1 tablespoon whole-grain Dijon mustard
6 tablespoons extra virgin olive oil
Kosher salt and freshly ground pepper
Combine the vinegar and mustard in a small bowl and whisk together. Slowly add the oil in a stream,

whisking to emulsify. Season with salt and pepper to taste.

Southern Caesar salad

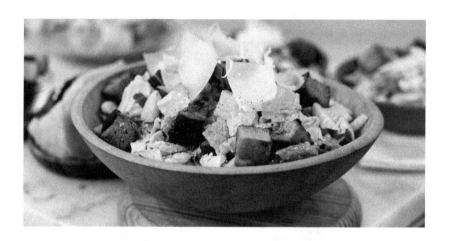

serves 6
ingredients:

One bag Hearts of Romaine
½ cup shredded Parmesan cheese
¼ pound country ham, sliced and cut into thin strips

Description:

In a large salad bowl, toss the Hearts of Romaine and
Parmesan cheese.
Add the seasoning of your choice and stir gently.
Divide the salad among individual plates.
Top with the sliced ham and grits croutons.

Serve immediately.

Confetti chip salad

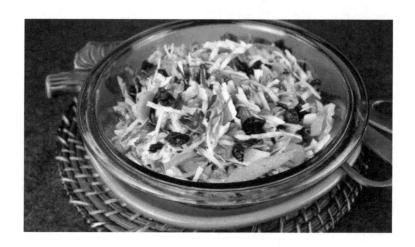

serves 4/6
ingredients:

1 bag Hearts of Romaine
½ red bell pepper, seeded and diced
½ yellow bell pepper, seeded and diced
1 ripe avocado, peeled and diced
1 cup of French fries

Description:

In a large salad bowl, put toss together the Hearts of
Romaine, red bell pepper, yellow bell pepper,
avocado, and vegetable chips.

Add dressing to taste and gently toss.
Serve immediately.

Dressing

¼ cup vegetable oil
¼ cup red wine vinegar
2 tablespoons sugar
1 tablespoon ketchup
Kosher salt and freshly ground pepper
A small bowl whisks together the oil, vinegar, sugar,
and ketchup until the sugar has dissolved.
Season with salt and pepper to taste.

Classic spinach salad

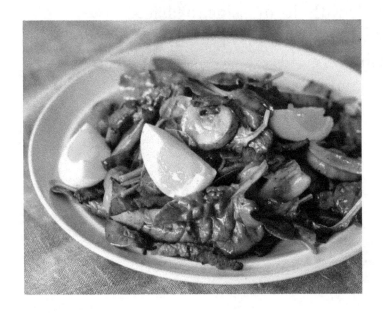

serves 6
ingredients:

salad
1 bag (6 ounces) Baby Spinach
½ red onion halved and thinly sliced
4 hard-boiled eggs, peeled and quartered
12 bacon slices, cooked and drained
6 button mushrooms, thinly sliced

Description:

Divide the Baby Spinach among individual plates.
Drizzle with the dressing to taste.
Top with the onion, eggs, bacon slices, and
mushrooms.
Serve immediately.

Grilled romaine

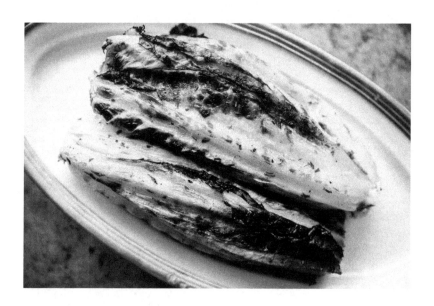

serves 6
ingredients:

green goddess dressing salad
1 bag (3 pack) Romaine Hearts
4 tablespoons extra-virgin olive oil
Kosher salt and freshly ground pepper
1 cup drained Mandarin orange slices
½ cup almond slices, toasted

Description:

Heat a clean grill to medium-high.
Cut the Romaine Hearts in half lengthwise.
Brush the romaine with the oil and season with salt and pepper to taste.
Grill, frequently turning, until slightly charred but not heated all the way through, about 5 minutes.
Place the grilled romaine on plates.
Drizzle with the dressing to taste and garnish with the Mandarin oranges and almond slices.
Serve immediately.

green goddess dressing

1 ripe avocado, peeled and diced
⅓ cup reduced-fat buttermilk
¼ cup fresh flat-leaf parsley leaves
2 tablespoons mayonnaise
2 tablespoons thinly sliced fresh chives
¼ teaspoon minced garlic
2 tablespoons freshly squeezed lemon juice
Kosher salt and freshly ground pepper
In a blender, purée the avocado, buttermilk, parsley, mayonnaise, chives, garlic, and lemon juice—season to taste with salt and pepper.

Pasta Rice and Couscous salad

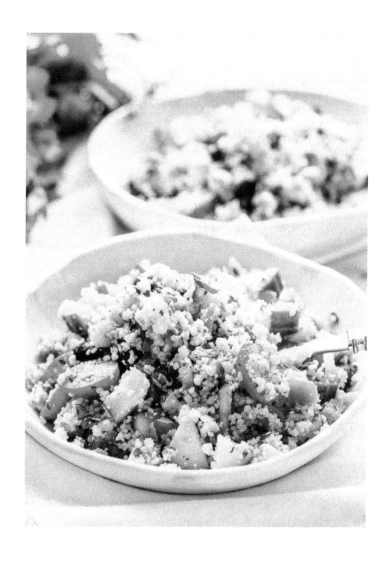

Lentil and tri-color pepper salad

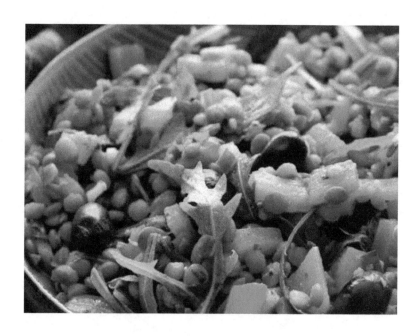

serves 6
ingredients:

1 yellow bell pepper
1 red bell pepper
1 orange bell pepper
1¼ cups lentils, rinsed and drained
3 cups water
½ yellow onion, peeled

1 garlic clove, peeled
Kosher salt and freshly ground pepper
½ red onion, thinly sliced
1 bag (6 ounces) Baby Spinach

Description:

To roast the peppers, heat a clean grill to high heat.
Lay the peppers on the grate and cook until well
charred.
Rotate the peppers a quarter turn and repeat until
each side is well charred.
Place the charred, hot peppers in a resealable bag.
Seal and steam until cooled to room temperature,
about 30 minutes.
Remove the peppers from the bag and, using a paper
towel, remove the skin. Gently pull the peppers apart
and remove and discard the seeds and stems. Thinly
slice the peppers.
In a large saucepan, combine the lentils the water,
yellow onion, and garlic and bring to a boil.
Reduce heat and simmer until lentils are tender but
still holding their shape, 20 to 25 minutes.
Drain the lentils and transfer to a large bowl; discard
the onion and garlic clove.
Pour the dressing over the warm lentils to taste and
stir to combine.
Season with salt and pepper to taste.
Set aside to cool to room temperature.

Stir the sliced peppers and red onion into the cooled lentils.
Divide the Baby Spinach among individual plates.
Top with a generous spoonful of lentils.
Serve immediately.

Brown rice, corn, and grilled vegetable salad

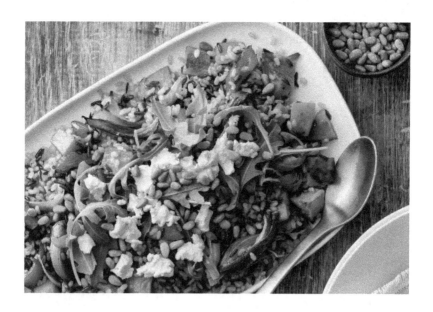

serves 6
ingredients:

1 zucchini, cut lengthwise and sliced into
¼-inch pieces
1 red bell pepper
1 red onion, cut into ½-inch slices
¼ cup extra-virgin olive oil
2 tablespoons soy sauce
2 ears corn, shucked

Kosher salt and freshly ground pepper
1 cup brown rice, cooked and cooled
1 bag Hearts of Romaine
Preheat a clean grill to medium.

Description:

In a large mixing bowl, toss the red onion, zucchini, red bell pepper, red onion, oil, and soy sauce until well coated. Marinate for 30 minutes.
Wrap the corn in aluminum foil and grill until tender, about 10 minutes.
When cool enough to handle, slice the corn kernels from the cob.
Put the corn kernels in a large salad bowl. Discard the cobs.
Season the vegetables with salt and pepper.
Transfer the vegetables, without excess marinade, to a grilling basket and grill until slightly charred, about 10 minutes per side.
Discard the marinade.
Combine the grilled vegetables with the corn. Let cool to room temperature.
Add the cooked rice and Hearts of Romaine to the vegetable mixture and toss.
Add the dressing to taste and toss to coat—season with salt and pepper to taste.

Curried rice and chickpea salad

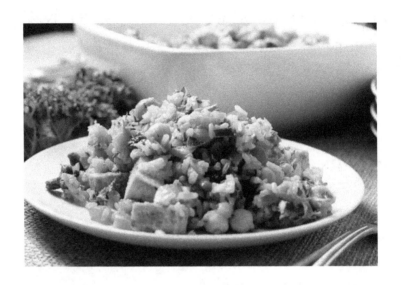

serves 4/6
ingredients:

1 cup brown rice, cooked and cooled
1 can chickpeas, rinsed and drained
1 bag shredded lettuce
½ red bell pepper, seeded and finely chopped
2 tablespoons slivered almonds, toasted
Kosher salt and freshly ground pepper

Description:

In a mixture large salad bowl, toss together the brown rice, chickpeas, shredded lettuce, red bell pepper, and almonds.
Add your preferred seasoning and toss gently.
Season with salt and pepper to taste.
Serve immediately.

curry dressing

¼ cup freshly squeezed orange juice
2 tablespoons white wine vinegar
3 tablespoons extra-virgin olive oil
½ teaspoon curry powder
In a plastic container, whisk together the curry, orange juice, vinegar, oil, powder until well combined.

Grilled portobello and Couscous salad

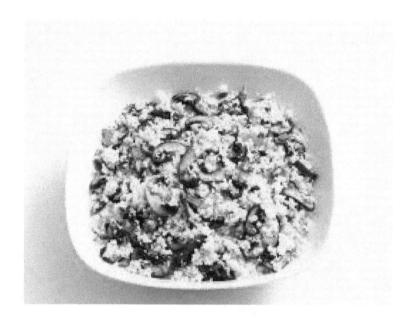

serves 8
ingredients:

¼ cup Red Wine Vinaigrette
Four large champignon caps, cleaned
2 tablespoons extra-virgin olive oil
Kosher salt and freshly ground pepper
1 cup plain couscous, cooked and cooled to room
temperature

1 carrot, peeled and finely diced
½ red bell pepper, seeded and finely diced
¼ red onion, finely diced
½ zucchini, finely diced
1 bag triple hearts

Description:

Prepare the Red Wine Vinaigrette.
Preheat a clean grill to medium-high.
Brush the champignon with oil and season with pepper and salt.
Grill until fork-tender, about 3 minutes per side. Set aside to cool to room temperature.
Cut into ½-inch slices.
In a large plastic salad bowl, toss together the prepared couscous, carrot, red bell pepper, onion, and zucchini.
Add the vinaigrette to taste, reserving some to drizzle over the triple hearts, and gently toss to coat.
Season with salt and pepper to taste.
Divide the Triple Hearts among the plates. Drizzle with the remaining vinaigrette. Top with a generous spoonful of the couscous mixture. Arrange the portobello slices across the top. Serve immediately.

Summer bean salad

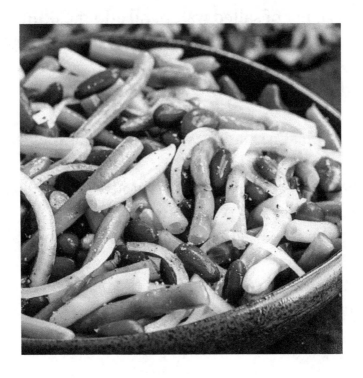

serves 6
ingredients:

¼ cup Lemon Vinaigrette
¾ pound yellow wax beans, stem ends trimmed
¾ cup cherry tomatoes halved crosswise
½ cup Kalamata olives pitted and halved
Kosher salt and freshly ground pepper
1 bag (5 ounces) Sweet Baby Greens
Prepare the Lemon Vinaigrette.

Description:

Put a large pot of salted water and add the beans, return to a boil, and cook for 3/5 minute until just tender.

Drain the beans and rinse with cold water until cooled.

In a large plastic salad bowl, toss together the beans, tomatoes, and olives.

Add the vinaigrette to taste and gently toss to coat.

Season with salt and pepper to taste.

Arrange the Sweet Baby Greens among individual plates.

Top with a generous spoonful of the bean salad.

Serve immediately.

Poultry Meat and Seafood salads

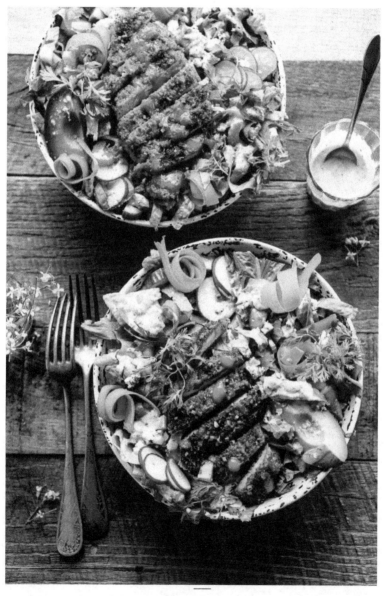

Chicken salad

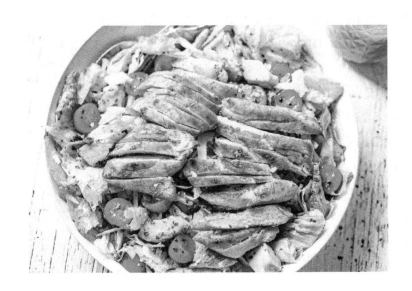

serves 8
ingredients:

½ cup Peanut Dressing
½ cup fresh snow peas
One bag spring mix
2 cups shredded cooked chicken
2 carrots, peeled and grated
¼ cup thinly sliced scallions
¼ cup fresh cilantro leaves
½ cup chopped roasted peanuts
2 limes, quartered, for garnish
Prepare the Peanut Dressing.

Description:

Boil salted water in a large pot and add the snow peas and cook until vibrant green and crisp-tender, 1 to 1½ minutes.

Drain the snow peas and immerse them in an ice-water bath to stop the cooking process.

Drain and place in a large plastic salad bowl.

Add the Spring Mix, chicken, carrots, scallions, cilantro, and peanuts, and toss.

Add seasoning as you prefer and toss gently to coat.

Garnish with lime wedges.

Serve immediately.

Margarita chicken salad

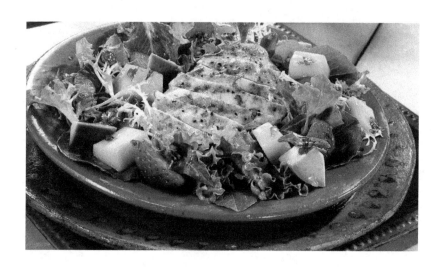

serves 4
ingredients:

½ cup freshly squeezed lime juice
¼ cup freshly squeezed orange juice
¼ cup tequila
1 tablespoon chili powder
½ fresh jalapeño, seeded and minced
2 small garlic cloves, minced
4 boneless, skinless chicken breasts
Kosher salt and freshly ground black pepper
1 bag (5 ounces) Spring Mix
½ cup toasted pepitas (pumpkin seeds)

½ cup dried cranberries
2 tangerines, peeled, sectioned, and seeded
1 cup crumbled Cojita Mexican cheese

Description:

In a medium-large steel bowl mix lime juice, orange juice, tequila, chili powder, jalapeño, and garlic.
Combine chicken breasts and stir to coat.
Cover and refrigerate for about 4 hours.
Heat a clean grill to medium-high. Remove the chicken from marinating, removing the excess, and season both sides with salt and pepper to taste.
Discard the marinade. Grill until well cooked about 6/ 8 minutes per sideand then remove the chicken breasts from the grill and let rest for 5/6 minutes.
Slice thinly against the grain.
In a large plastic salad bowl, toss together the spring mix, pepitas, cranberries, tangerine sections, and cheese.
Add the dressing to taste and gently toss to coat.
Divide the salad among individual plates.
Top with the sliced chicken.
Serve immediately.

Jalapeño chicken salad

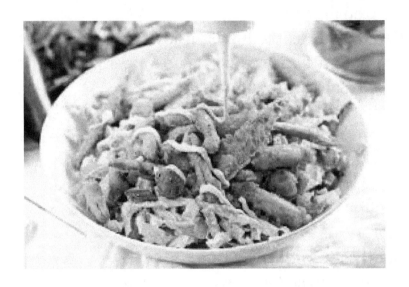

serves 4/6
ingredients:

3 skinless, boneless chicken breasts
4 tablespoons mayonnaise
2 teaspoons finely grated lime zest
2 tablespoons finely chopped shallots
2 tablespoons finely chopped seeded red bell pepper
1 teaspoon chopped seeded fresh jalapeño
1 ripe avocado, peeled and diced
Kosher salt and freshly ground pepper
1 bag Riviera™ Blend

Description:

Bring a large saucepan of salted water to boil. Add the chicken breasts.
Reduce the heat to medium-low, cover, and gently simmer until the chicken is no longer pink in the middle, about 12 minutes.
Transfer to a plate to cool.
When cold cut the chicken into ½ inch pieces cubes.
In a large plastic bowl, combine the mayonnaise, lime zest, shallots, red bell pepper, and jalapeño.
Fold the chicken into the mayonnaise mixture to coat.
Gently stir in the diced avocado.
Season with salt and pepper to taste.
Place the Riviera Blend in a large salad bowl. Add the dressing.
Divide the salad among individual plates. Top with a generous scoop of the chicken salad.

avocado vinaigrette

3 tablespoons vegetable oil
5 tablespoons freshly squeezed lime juice
¼ cup sour cream
1 ripe avocado, peeled and diced
2 to 3 tablespoons room temperature water
Kosher salt and freshly ground pepper

Place the oil, lime juice, sour cream, and avocado in a blender.
Blend until smooth.
Thin with room temperature water as needed.
Season with salt and pepper to taste.

Fried chicken salad

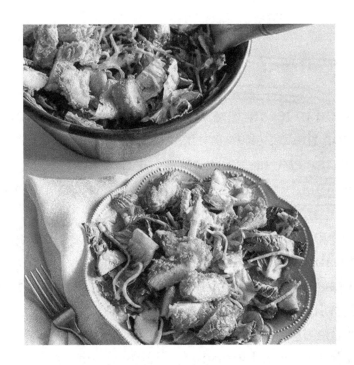

serves 6/8
ingredients:

One tablespoon vegetable oil
3 skinless, boneless chicken breasts, cut into
⅓-inch cubes
Kosher salt and freshly ground pepper
¼ cup fresh basil leaves, thinly sliced
¼ cup chopped roasted peanuts
One tablespoon peeled and grated fresh ginger

1 bag Baby Spinach
½ bag Broccoli Slaw
1 cucumber
1 red bell pepper

Description:

Heat oil in a saucepan over medium-high heat.
Season the chicken with salt and pepper.
Place the chicken and cook for 6/8 minutes,
occasionally stirring, until well browned and no
longer pink in the middle.
Remove the heat and put the basil, peanuts, ginger,
and half of the dressing. Toss to coat.
In a large plastic salad bowl, toss the Baby Spinach,
Broccoli Slaw, cucumber, and red bell pepper.
Add the dressing to taste.
Divide the salad among individual plates.
Top with the warm chicken mixture.
Serve immediately.

Southern fried chicken salad

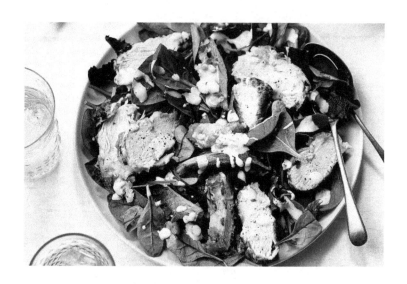

serves6
ingredients:

3 skinless, boneless chicken breasts
12 chicken tenders
1½ cups reduced-fat buttermilk
1½ cups all-purpose flour
1 tablespoon kosher salt
1 tablespoon freshly ground black pepper
1-quart vegetable oil for frying
2 bags american blend
8 hard-boiled eggs, peeled and halved
2 tomatoes, cut into eight wedges each

8 baby dill pickles, halved lengthwise

Description:

Place the chicken tenders in a large bowl and add the buttermilk and toss to coat.
Cover, refrigerate and marinate for up to 12 hours.
Combine the flour, salt, and pepper in a large bowl.
Working in small batches, remove the chicken from the buttermilk, shaking off the excess, and place in the flour mixture.
Pat gently to evenly coat.
Discard the marinade.
Pour 1-inch of oil in the bottom of a heavy stockpot. Heat to medium-high heat or until a deep-fry or candy thermometer registers 360°F. Working in small batches, carefully place the chicken tenders in the hot oil and fry until the chicken is well browned inside, about 15 minutes. Allow the oil to return to 360°F between batches.
Place the cooked chicken strips on a rack to drain.
Divide the American Blend among individual plates. Arrange the eggs, tomato wedges, dill pickles, and fried chicken on top. Drizzle with the dressing to taste.
Serve immediately.

Chicken tostada salad

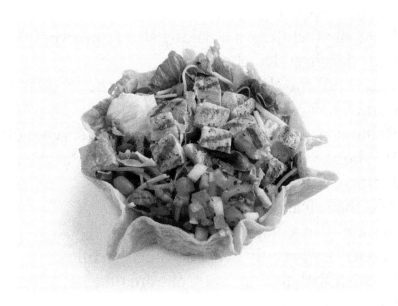

serves 6
ingredients:

4 8-inch round flour tortillas
¾ cup coarsely shredded pepper Jack cheese
1 bag shredded lettuce
2 cups shredded cooked chicken
¼ cup fresh cilantro leaves, coarsely chopped
1 cup jarred green salsa
Kosher salt and freshly ground pepper
1 large tomato, diced
¼ cup sour cream

Description:

Preheat oven to 385°F.
Place the tortillas on a baking sheet and evenly cover with the shredded cheese.
Bake until the cheese is melted and the tortillas are crunchy, about 7/8 min.
Remove pan from oven and transfer to serving plates.
In a large salad bowl, toss together the Shredded Lettuce, chicken, and cilantro.
Add the salsa.
Season with salt and pepper to taste.
Spoon salad evenly over the warm tortillas.
Garnish with tomato and sour cream.
Serve immediately.

Chicken Florentine salad

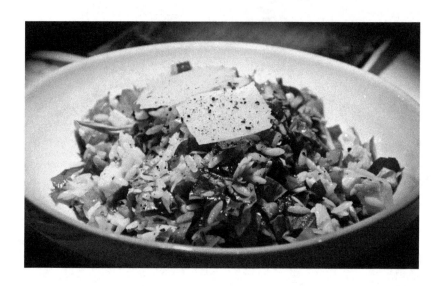

serves 6
ingredients:

Four skinless, boneless chicken breasts, grilled,
cooled, and thinly sliced
½ cup pine nuts, toasted
¼ cup sliced black olives (available in a can)
3 tablespoons capers, drained and rinsed
1 bag (6 ounces) Baby Spinach
1 cup cooked orzo, drained, rinsed, and cooled to
room temperature

Description:

In a large plastic salad bowl, toss together the sliced chicken, pine nuts, black olives, capers, Baby Spinach, and orzo.

Add the lemon vinaigrette to taste and gently toss to coat.

Serve immediately.

lemon-parmesan vinaigrette

2 tablespoons freshly squeezed lemon juice

1 teaspoon Dijon mustard

½ small garlic clove, mashed to a paste or minced

¼ cup extra virgin olive oil

1 tablespoon finely shredded Parmesan cheese

Kosher salt and freshly ground pepper

In a small plastic bowl, whisk together the lemon juice, mustard, and garlic. Slowly add the oil in a steady stream, whisking to emulsify. Stir in the cheese.

Season with salt and pepper to taste.

Taco salad

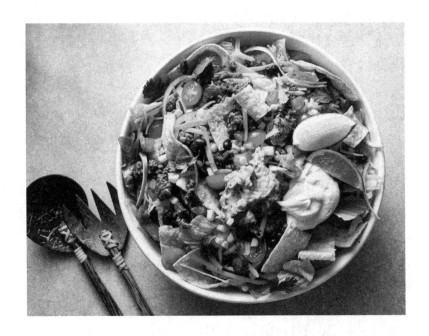

serves 4
ingredients:

1 pound ground beef
1 package (1.25 ounces) taco seasoning
2 bags (8 ounces each) Shredded Lettuce
15 ounces kidney beans, rinsed and drained
2 tomatoes, diced
2 ripe avocados, peeled and diced
1 small white onion, diced
1½ cups shredded sharp Cheddar cheese

2 cups tortilla chips
1½ cups salsa
1 cup sour cream
¼ cup pickled sliced jalapeños (optional)

Description:

Brown the ground beef in a frying pan over medium heat and add the taco seasoning package and mix well. Set aside.

Divide the Shredded Lettuce among individual bowls. Spoon a generous serving of the cooked beef in the center of each bed of lettuce.

Add the beans, tomatoes, avocados, white onion, and cheese.

Tuck the tortilla chips into the sides of the salad.

Generously drizzle with the salsa to taste.

Garnish with the sour cream and jalapeños, if desired.

Serve immediately.

Thai beef salad

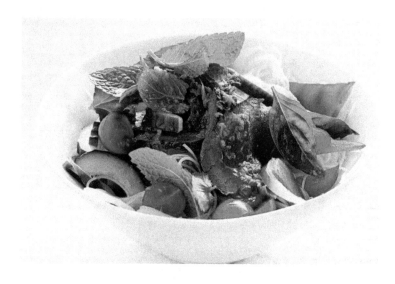

serves 4/6
ingredients:

1 pound flank steak
Kosher salt and freshly ground black pepper
1 cucumber, peeled, cut lengthwise without removing
the seeds
2 shallots, thinly sliced crosswise into rings
1 tablespoon coarsely chopped fresh cilantro
1 tablespoon coarsely chopped fresh mint
1 bag (10 ounces) Hearts of Romaine
½ cup coarsely chopped unsalted, roasted peanuts

Description:

Place the steak in a shallow dish.
Pour ⅓ of the dressing over the steak, turning to coat.
Cover, refrigerate and marinate 1 to 2 hours. Reserve
the remaining sauce for use later.
Heat a clean grill to medium-high.
Remove the steak from the marinade,shaking off
excess.
Discard the marinade. Season both sides of the steak
with pepper and salt.
Grill, turning as needed, until medium-rare, 4 to 6
minutes per side, or until the desired doneness.
Remove the steak from the grill after few minutes and
set it aside to rest for 5 to 10 minutes before slicing.
Slice thinly against the grain.
In a large plastic bowl, toss together the sliced steak,
cucumber, shallots, cilantro, and mint.
Add the remaining dressing to taste, reserving some
to drizzle on top of the hearts of romaine, and gently
toss.
Divide the hearts of romaine equally among the
plates and drizzle with the remaining dressing.
Generously spoon the warm steak mixture over the
beds of lettuce.
Garnish with the chopped peanuts.
Serve immediately.

dressing and marinade

¼ cup freshly squeezed lime juice
¼ cup fish sauce
2 teaspoons dark brown sugar
¼ teaspoon red pepper flakes
A small plastic bowl whisks together the lime juice, fish sauce, brown sugar, and red pepper flakes until the sugar has dissolved.

Grilled pork tenderloin salad

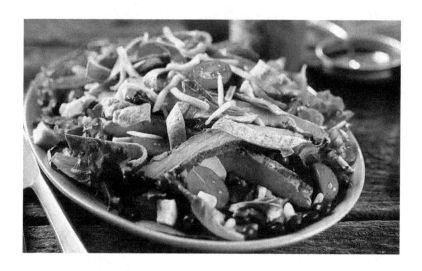

serves 6/8
ingredients:

½ cup apricot preserves
2 tablespoons white wine vinegar
1 tablespoon Dijon mustard
½ teaspoon ground ginger
1 to 1¼ pounds pork
Kosher salt and freshly ground pepper
1 bag (10 ounces) European Blend
½ cup drained and sliced canned or jarred apricot halves
½ cup dried cherries

¼ cup thinly sliced scallions
¼ cup sliced almonds, toasted

Description:

Heat a clean grill to medium-high.
To prepare an apricot glaze, whisk together the apricot preserves, vinegar,mustard, and ginger in a small bowl.
Season the pork with pepper and salt.
Grill over medium-high heat until well-done, brushing with the apricot glaze the last 2 minutes of cooking per side, 5 to 6 minutes per side.
Remove the tenderloin from the heat and set it aside to rest for 5 to 10 minutes before slicing. Slice thinly across the grain.
In a large plastic salad bowl, toss together the European Blend, apricots, cherries, scallions, and almonds.
Add the vinaigrette and gently toss. Divide equally among individual plates.
Arrange the pork tenderloin slices on top of the salad. Serve immediately.

apricot balsamic vinaigrette

2 tablespoons balsamic vinegar
½ teaspoon yellow or Dijon mustard Dash of soy sauce

1 garlic clove, minced
1 teaspoon apricot preserves
¼ cup extra-virgin olive oil
Kosher salt and freshly ground pepper
In a small plastic bowl, whisk together the vinegar,
mustard, soy sauce, garlic, and apricot preserves.
Slowly add the oil in a stream, whisking to emulsify.
Season with salt and pepper to taste.

Grilled lamb and tabbouleh salad

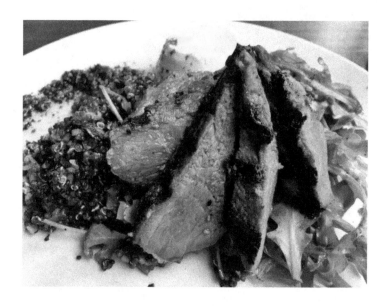

serves 4
ingredients:

1 pound trimmed boneless leg of lamb
Kosher salt and freshly ground pepper
1 red onion, sliced into rings
2 tablespoons extra-virgin olive oil
1 bag (6 ounces) Baby Spinach
1 cup prepared tabbouleh
½ cup crumbled feta cheese

Description:

Preheat a clean grill to medium-high.
Butterfly the lamb by cutting horizontally through the thickest part of the meat, leaving about 1 inch still attached. Open flat and season with salt and pepper.
Place the sliced onion in a medium bowl and drizzle with the oil; toss to coat.
Place the lamb and onion slices on the prepared grill. Grill the lamb until medium-rare, about 8 minutes per side, or until the desired doneness. Grill the onion slices in a grilling basket until tender, about 5 minutes per side.
Set the lamb aside to rest for 5 to 10 minutes before slicing.
Thinly slice the lamb diagonally across the grain.
Place the Baby Spinach in a large salad bowl. Add the dressing to taste and gently toss. Divide the salad among individual plates. Spoon about ¼ cup of the tabbouleh over the top.
Arrange the lamb slices and onions over each salad. Garnish with the crumbled feta cheese.
Serve immediately.

Vinaigrette

2 tablespoons red wine vinegar
1 tablespoon freshly squeezed lemon juice
6 tablespoons extra-virgin olive oil

Kosher salt and freshly ground pepper
In a small plastic bowl whisk together the vinegar and lemon juice.
Slowly add the oil in a stream, whisking to emulsify.
Season with salt and pepper to taste.

Fajita salad

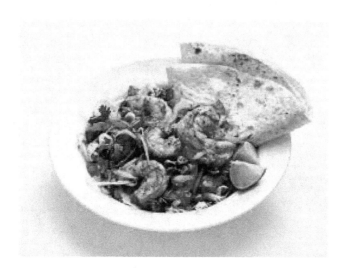

serves 4
ingredients:

2 tablespoons freshly squeezed lime juice
3 tablespoons tequila
1 tablespoon ground cumin
1 garlic clove, minced
1½ pounds flank steak, cut across the grain into ½-inch thick slices
4 8-inch round flour tortillas
Kosher salt and freshly ground pepper
1 tablespoon olive oil
1 red bell pepper
1 green bell pepper

½ red onion halved and thinly sliced
1 bag (10 ounces) Leafy Romaine

Description:

In a small plastic bowl, whisk together the lime juice, tequila, cumin, and garlic.

Pour the marinade over the flank steak, cover, and marinate 1 hour.

Preheat the oven to 375°F. In ovenproof bowls similar in size to your serving dish, place the tortillas.

Press down on each tortilla until it is the shape of a bowl.

Bake until golden brown and crisp for 12/15 minutes.

Remove from the oven and let cool to room temperature.

Remove steak from marinade by removing the excess. Discard the marinade. Season with salt and pepper.

In a baking dish over high heat, warm the oil until a few water droplets sizzle in the pan. Add the steak and sear, often stirring, until well browned, 4 minutes.

Add the red bell pepper, green bell pepper, and onion and cook, often stirring, until the vegetables are golden brown, and the steak is cooked to desired doneness, about four more minutes for medium-rare.

Place the Leafy Romaine in a large salad bowl. Add the vinaigrette to taste and gently toss—season with salt and pepper to taste.

Place the tortilla "bowls" on individual dishes. Fill with the Leafy Romaine.
Top with the warm fajita mixture. Garnish with the Pico de Gallo.
Serve immediately.

pico de gallo
½ small white onion, finely diced
1 large tomato, seeded and diced
½ green bell pepper, seeded and finely diced
1 teaspoon chopped seeded fresh jalapeño
3 tablespoons freshly squeezed lime juice
1 tablespoon extra-virgin olive oil
Kosher salt and freshly ground pepper
In a medium bowl, toss together the onion, tomato, bell pepper, jalapeño, lime
juice, and oil. Season with salt and pepper to taste.

Seared salmon over mixed greens

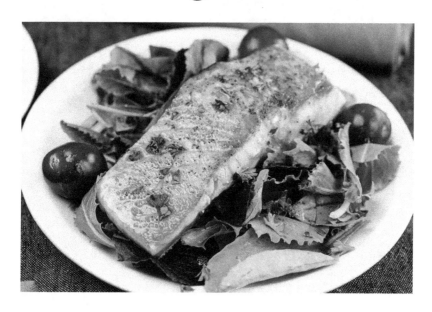

serves 4
ingredients:

4 boneless salmon fillets
Kosher salt and freshly ground pepper
2 tablespoons extra-virgin olive oil
1 bag (5 ounces) Spring Mix
½ cup dried cranberries
¼ cup thinly sliced scallions
½ cup crumbled feta cheese

Description:

Sprinkle the salmon with pepper and salt then heat the oil in a large skillet over medium heat. Cook the salmon for about 4 minutes, skin side up, until the flesh is nicely browned and comes away from the pan easily. Turn salmon fillets over and cook until medium., about five more minutes, or until the desired doneness.

In the meantime that the salmon finishes cooking, mix the spring mix with the blueberries mix with the cranberries, scallions, feta cheese, and ¾ cup pecans in a large salad bowl. Reserve the remaining pecans for another use. Add the vinaigrette, reserving some to drizzle on top of the fish, and gently toss. Season with salt and pepper to taste.

Place the salmon fillets on top of the salad spread out on a serving platter.

Wet the salmon well with the vinaigrette. Serve immediately.

Tuna niçoise

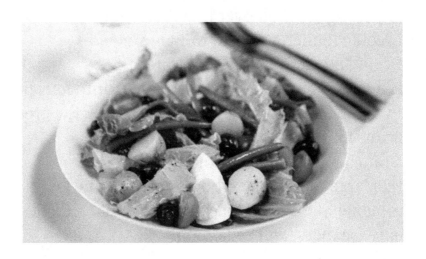

serves 6
ingredients:

½ cup Vinaigrette
8 small red new potatoes
¼ pound fresh green beans, trimmed
1 bag leafy romaine
6 ounces tuna, drained and flaked
2 radishes, trimmed and thinly sliced
½ cup Niçoise olives pitted
¼ cup capers drained and rinsed
½ red onion halved and thinly sliced

Description:

Place all the potatoes in a large pot of salted water
and bring to a boil over high heat and cook until they
become tender about 10 to 15 minutes.
Drain and rinse under cold water.
When they are cold, cut the potatoes into four parts.
In another pot of hot, salted water, cook the green
beans for about 3/4 minutes.
Drain and rinse under cold water.
In a large plastic salad bowl, combine the leafy
romaine, potatoes, haricots verts, tuna, radishes,
olives, capers, and red onion.
Add the vinaigrette.
Serve immediately.

Salmon and asparagus salad

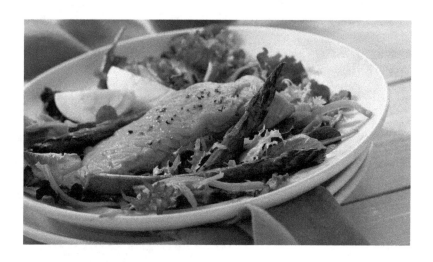

serves 6
ingredients:

4 boneless salmon fillets
Kosher salt and freshly ground pepper
1 tablespoon olive oil
½ bunch (about ½ pound) asparagus spears,
trimmed
1 bag Hearts of Romaine
¾ cup cherry tomatoes halved

Description:

Preheat oven to 380°F and place the salmon fillets, skin side down, in a shallow baking dish.

Season with salt and pepper to taste.

Drizzle with olive oil.

Bake for about 15/18 minutes until cooked through.

Remove from oven and allow to cool. Once cold, gently shred with a fork, removing the skin.

Cut the trimmed asparagus spears into 1½-inch pieces.

In a pot, bring salted water to a boil and then add the asparagus and cook until vibrant green and crisp-tender, 1 to 1½ minutes.

Drain asparagus and soak in cold water to stop cooking, then drain and place in a large salad bowl.

Add the Hearts of Romaine, salmon, and cherry tomatoes.

Add the vinaigrette and serve immediately.

pesto vinaigrette
fresh basil leaves
1 small clove of chopped garlic
1 tablespoon grated parmesan cheese
1 tablespoon of toasted pine nuts
1½ tablespoons red wine vinegar
½ cup extra-virgin olive oil
Kosher salt and freshly ground pepper

In a food processor or blender, pureé the basil, garlic, Parmesan cheese, pine nuts, vinegar, and oil until smooth. Season with salt and pepper to taste.

Pancetta-wrapped scallops

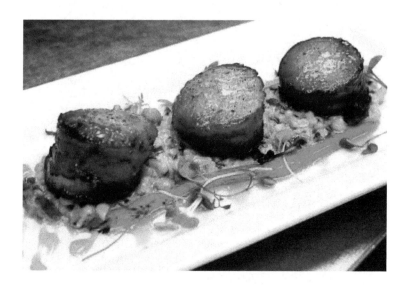

serves 4/6
ingredients:

12 large sea scallops
½ pound pancetta, thinly sliced (at least 12 slices)
5 ounces Spring mix
Kosher salt and freshly ground pepper

Description:

Rinse the scallops, pat dry, and place in a large bowl.
Pour half the vinaigrette over the scallops; toss to
coat. Reserve the remaining vinaigrette for the salad.

Cover, refrigerate and let the scallops marinate for 1 hour.

Preheat the oven to 375°F.

Remove the scallops from the marinade and wrap each scallop with one slice of pancetta. Place the scallops 1-inch apart on an ungreased rimmed baking pan.

Bake until the pancetta is crispy, about 10 minutes. Place the Spring Mix in a large salad bowl. Add the reserved vinaigrette to taste and gently toss. Season with salt and pepper to taste. Divide the salad equally among the plates. Arrange the scallops, equally divided, on the plates.

Serve immediately.

rosemary-lemon vinaigrette

1 teaspoon finely grated lemon zest

¼ cup freshly squeezed lemon juice

½ cup extra-virgin olive oil

Four tablespoons minced fresh rosemary

In a small plastic bowl, whisk together the lemon zest and lemon juice.

Slowly add the oil in a steady stream, whisking to emulsify. Stir in the rosemary.

Shrimp stir-fry salad

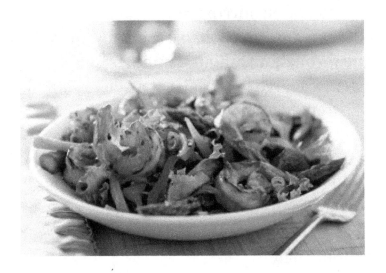

serves 6
ingredients:

1 tablespoon peanut oil
1 tablespoon red Thai curry paste
1 pound of shrimps, without tail and skin and cut in half
12 cherry tomatoes, halved
¼ cup scallions, sliced ½-inch long on the diagonal
1 bag Asian Salad Blend

Description:

In a wok over medium-high heat, warm the oil and curry paste, often stirring, until fragrant.
Add the shrimp and cook, occasionally stirring, until opaque throughout, about 3 minutes.
Transfer to a large bowl and set aside to cool, then add the tomatoes and the scallions to the shrimp.
Add half the dressing to taste and gently toss.
Place the Asian salad mixture in a large salad bowl, then add the remaining dressing and toss gently.
Divide the Asian salad blend among the plates.
Generously spoon the shrimp mixture on top.
Serve immediately.

Thai dressing

2 tablespoons dark brown sugar
1 teaspoon finely grated lime zest
¼ cup freshly squeezed lime juice
1 Thai chili pepper, seeded, and minced
2 lemongrass stalks, very thinly sliced
1 shallot, thinly sliced
3 tablespoons finely chopped fresh cilantro
In a small plastic bowl, whisk together the brown sugar, lime zest, and lime juice until the sugar is dissolved. Stir in the chili pepper, lemongrass, shallot, and cilantro.

Lobster salad

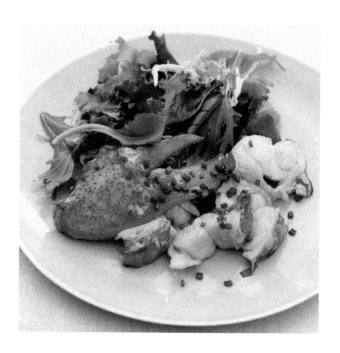

serves 6
ingredients:

Two 1-pound lobsters freshly cooked and shelled
¼ cup thinly sliced celery
½ red bell pepper, seeded and diced
1 tablespoon minced fresh basil
1 tablespoon minced fresh mint
1 bag (7 ounces) Riviera™ Blend, torn into small pieces

Description:

Cut the lobster meat into ½-inch pieces.
Place the lobster meat in a large salad bowl. Add the celery, red bell pepper, basil, mint, and the Riviera Blend.
Add the vinaigrette and gently toss then serve immediately.

grapefruit vinaigrette
4 tablespoons freshly squeezed grapefruit juice
2 tablespoons freshly squeezed lime juice
1 tablespoon minced shallot
2 tablespoons canola oil
Kosher salt and freshly ground pepper
In a small plastic bowl, whisk together the grapefruit juice, lime juice, shallot, and oil until well combined—season with salt and pepper to taste.

Spanish shrimp, orange, and olive salad

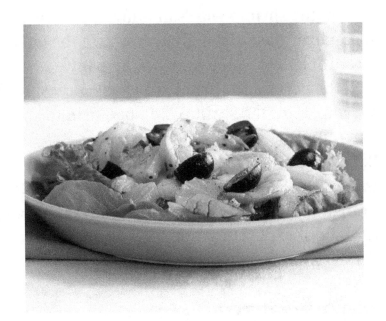

serves 6
ingredients:

¾ pound shrimp tails removed, and deveined
Kosher salt and freshly ground pepper
2 tablespoons olive oil
1 small garlic clove, minced
3 oranges, peeled and thinly sliced
½ cup sliced Spanish green olives

1 teaspoon finely grated orange peel
5 ounces Baby Arugula

Description:

Season the shrimp with salt and pepper. In a large skillet over medium-high heat, warm the oil until a few droplets of water sizzle in the pan.
Add the garlic and shrimp and cook, occasionally stirring, until the shrimp are opaque in the center, 3 to 5 minutes.
Set aside and cool to room temperature.
In a large plastic bowl, toss together the shrimp, orange slices, olives, orange peel, and Baby Arugula. Add the sherry vinaigrette to taste and gently toss. Serve immediately.

sherry vinaigrette

1 shallot, minced
1 teaspoon Dijon mustard
2 tablespoons sherry wine vinegar
6 tablespoons extra-virgin olive oil
Kosher salt and freshly ground pepper
In a small plastic bowl, whisk together the shallot, mustard, and vinegar. Slowly add the olive oil in a stream, whisking to emulsify—season with salt and pepper to taste.

Maryland crab cake salad

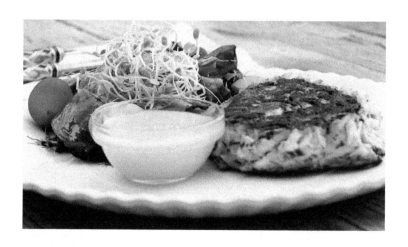

serves 6
ingredients:

1 pound jumbo lump crabmeat
1 egg, cracked into a small bowl
1 tablespoon mayonnaise
1 teaspoon Dijon mustard
1 teaspoon Worcestershire sauce
2 tablespoons minced fresh parsley
Kosher salt and freshly ground pepper
½ red bell pepper, seeded and finely diced
1 shallot, minced
3 tablespoons breadcrumbs
¼ cup White Balsamic Vinaigrette

Vegetable oil for frying
8 ounces Mediterranean Blend

Description:

Gather the crabmeat from the shell and in a plastic
bowl beat the egg the mayonnaise, mustard,
Worcestershire sauce and parsley. Season to taste
with salt and pepper.
Gently fold the crabmeat, red bell pepper, shallot, and
breadcrumbs into the egg mixture. Shape into eight
crab cakes then cover with plastic wrap and
refrigerate for 30 minutes.
Prepare the White Balsamic Vinaigrette.
Fill a large skillet with vegetable oil and heat the oil
over high heat.
Fry the cakes until golden brown, about 5 minutes
per side.
Remove from pan and set aside; keep warm.
Divide the Mediterranean Blend among individual
plates. Drizzle the dressing over the salad to taste.
Arrange the crab cakes on the salad.
Garnish with a generous spoonful of caper
remoulade.
Serve immediately.

caper remoulade

¼ cup mayonnaise
¼ cup sour cream
2 tablespoons freshly squeezed lemon juice
4 tablespoons capers, drained and rinsed
Kosher salt and freshly ground pepper
In a small plastic bowl, whisk together the
mayonnaise, sour cream, and lemon juice.
Stir in the capers—season with salt and pepper to
taste.

Vegetables and Fruits salad

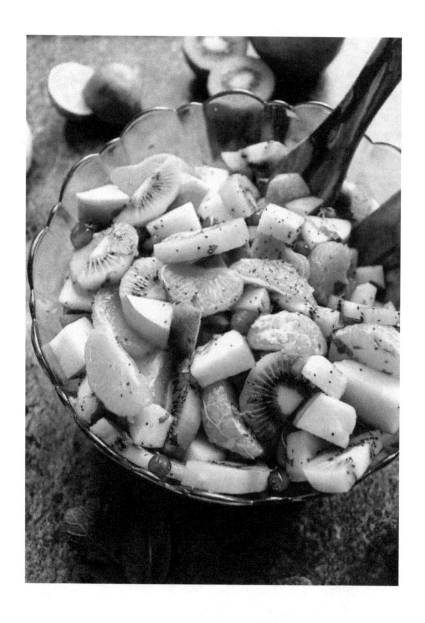

Warm potato salad

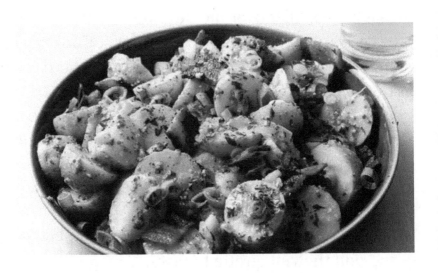

serves 6
ingredients:

¼ cup Garlic Vinaigrette
1 pound small fingerling potatoes, cleaned
3 tablespoons extra-virgin olive oil
½ thin baguette (8 ounces), thinly sliced
8 slices of bacon
1 bag (8 ounces) Field Greens

Description:

Prepare the Garlic Vinaigrette.
Cook all the potatoes in a large pot of salted water.

Reduce the heat and simmer until the potatoes are fork-tender, eight to10 minutes then drain and keep warm.

In a large skillet over medium heat, warm the oil until a few water droplets sizzle in the pan. Cook the bread slices, often stirring, until golden brown and crisp, about 5 min.

Using a slotted spoon and transfer croutons to a plate with paper towels to drain. In the same pan, cook the bacon(3 or4minutes), turning as needed, until crisp. Place bacon on a plate with sheets of paper towels and keep warm.

Place the warm potatoes in a large salad plastic bowl and add the vinaigrette to taste.

Toss to coat well. Add the Field Greens and toss gently. Tear the bacon into 1- inch pieces and add to the salad along with the croutons. Serve immediately.

Greek salad

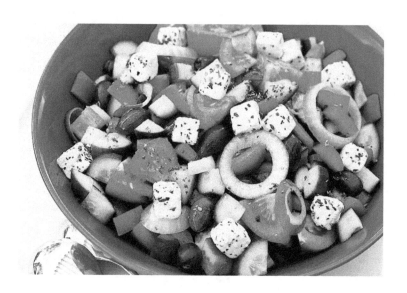

serves 6/8
ingredients:

1 bag (8 ounces) Mediterranean Blend
2 Roma tomatoes, diced
½ red onion, thinly sliced
½ green bell pepper seedless and thinly sliced
½ red bell pepper, seedless and thinly sliced
1 small cucumber, thinly sliced
¼ cup thinly sliced scallions
½ cup Kalamata olives pitted
⅓ cup Feta cheese

Description:

In a large plastic salad bowl, toss together the Mediterranean blend, tomatoes, red onion, green and red bell peppers, cucumber, and scallions. Add the dressing and toss gently and combine the salad with the olives and feta cheese. Serve immediately.

greek vinaigrette

3 tablespoons red wine vinegar
1 teaspoon freshly squeezed lemon juice
1 teaspoon dried oregano
1 small garlic clove, mashed to a paste (see page 230 for instructions)
or minced
6 tablespoons extra-virgin olive oil
Kosher salt and freshly ground pepper
In a small plastic, bowl whisks together the vinegar, lemon juice, oregano, and garlic.
Slowly add the oil in a steady stream, whisking until emulsified—season to taste with salt and pepper.

Layered chop salad

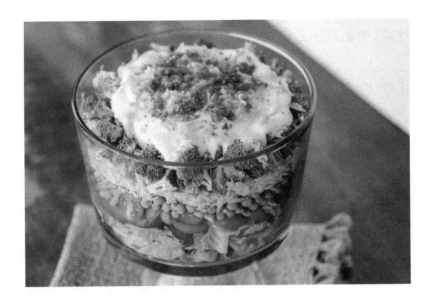

serves 10
ingredients:

1¼ cups Buttermilk Garlic Dressing
1 bag frozen green peas, thawed
1 can (15 ounces) chickpeas, rinsed and drained
1 package (8 ounces) Shredded Lettuce
2 red bell peppers, seeded and diced
1 bunch scallions, thinly sliced
1 bag (10 ounces) Shredded Carrots
4 cucumbers, halved lengthwise, seeded, and diced

4 Roma tomatoes, quartered lengthwise, seeded, and diced
1 can (6 ounces) fried onions

Description:

Prepare the Buttermilk Garlic Dressing.
In a large glass bowl, layer the green peas, chickpeas, Shredded Lettuce, red bell peppers, scallions, carrots, cucumbers, and tomatoes.
Pour the dressing over the top and set aside until the layers are soaked through about 5 minutes. Just before serving, top with the fried onions.

Panzanella

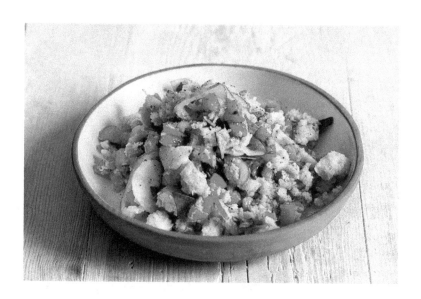

serves 10
ingredients:

1 ripe tomato, cut into 1-inch pieces
1 small cucumber
1 red bell pepper, seeded and cut into 1-inch pieces
1 yellow bell pepper, seeded and cut into
1-inch pieces
½ red onion halved and thinly sliced
10 large basil leaves, sliced into thin strips
1 bag (7 ounces) Riviera™ Blend

Description:

In a large plastic salad bowl, toss together the tomato, cucumber, red bell pepper, yellow bell pepper, red onion, basil, and the Riviera Blend.

Add the croutons and the vinaigrette to taste. Toss gently. Set aside to allow the croutons to soak up the vinaigrette, 10 to 20 minutes.

croutons

2 tablespoons extra-virgin olive oil
½ small loaf of French or Italian country bread (15 ounces), cut into 1-inch cubes.

In a large sauté pan over medium heat, warm the oil until a few water droplets sizzle in the pan. Add the bread and cook, stirring as needed, until golden brown, about 4 minutes. Using a slotted spoon, transfer croutons to a paper towel–lined plate to drain. Cool to room temperature.

Hearts of palm salad

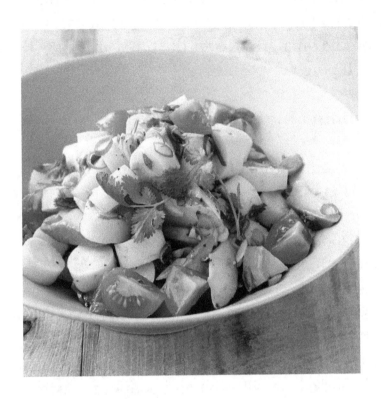

serves 6
ingredients:

1 bag (5 ounces) Sweet Baby Lettuces
14 ounces hearts of palm sliced
1 red pepper, seeded and finely diced

Description:

Divide the Sweet Baby Lettuces equally among individual plates. Arrange the hearts of palm on top. Spoon the vinaigrette over the top. Garnish with the red bell pepper.

red onion vinaigrette

2 tablespoons white balsamic vinegar
1 tablespoon whole-grain Dijon mustard
1 garlic clove, minced
6 tablespoons extra-virgin olive oil
Kosher salt and freshly ground pepper
½ medium red onion, thinly sliced into rings
In a small plastic bowl, whisk together the vinegar, mustard, and garlic.
Slowly add the oil in a steady stream, whisking to emulsify. Season with salt and pepper to taste.
Add the onion and toss to coat.
Refrigerate for 30 minutes to marinate the onion.

Grilled vegetable salad

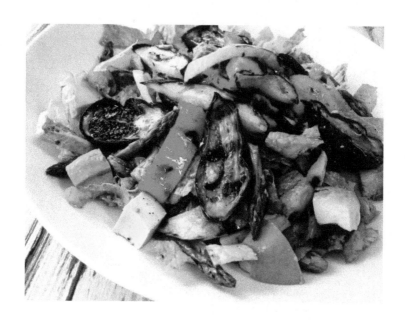

serves 6
ingredients:

1 zucchini, cut
1 yellow squash, cut
1 small eggplant, cut into 1-inch cubes
1 red bell bell pepper, seeded and cut into 1-inch
1 red onion
1 tablespoon dried Italian seasoning
Kosher salt and freshly ground pepper
1 bag (10 ounces) Hearts of Romaine Parmesan
shavings for garnish

Description:

Preheat a clean grill to medium.

In a large plastic bowl, toss the zucchini, squash, eggplant, red bell pepper, red onion, Italian seasoning, and ¼ cup of the vinaigrette until well coated. Marinate for 30 minutes.

Season the vegetables with salt and pepper. Transfer the vegetables, shaking off the excess marinade, to a grill basket and grill until slightly charred, about 10 minutes per side. Place in a large salad bowl and let cool to room temperature.

Add the Hearts of Romaine to the cooked vegetables and toss. Add the remaining vinaigrette to taste and gently toss. Divide among individual plates.

Garnish with the Parmesan cheese shavings.

Serve immediately.

balsamic vinaigrette

¼ cup balsamic vinegar

¾ cup extra-virgin olive oil

Kosher salt and freshly ground pepper

Place the vinegar in a small bowl. Slowly add the oil in a steady stream, whisking to emulsify. Season with salt and pepper to taste.

Mango, avocado, and cilantro salad

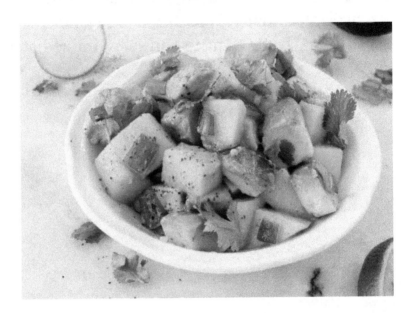

serves 4
ingredients:

¼ cup White Balsamic Vinaigrette
1 bag (5 ounces) Spring Mix
2 ripe avocados, peeled and diced
1 mango, seeded, diced, and peeled
½ red onion, finely diced
½ cup fresh cilantro leaves

Description:

Prepare the White Balsamic Vinaigrette.
In a large plastic salad bowl, toss together the Spring
Mix, avocados, mango, red onion, and cilantro.
Add the vinaigrette to taste and serve immediately.

English farmhouse salad

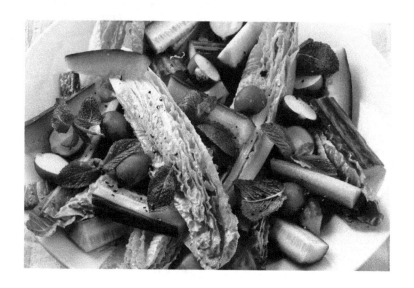

serves 4
ingredients.

1 apple, cored and thinly sliced
1 tablespoon canola or vegetable oil
1 bag (5 ounces) Spring Mix
½ cup walnuts, toasted and cooled
½ cup crumbled Stilton blue cheese

Description:

Preheat a clean grill pan to medium-low.
In a large steel bowl, toss the apple slices with the oil until well coated. Place the apple slices in a grilling basket and grill until just softened, about 2 minutes per side.
In a large plastic salad bowl, toss the Spring Mix, walnuts, and Stilton cheese. Add the vinaigrette to taste and gently toss. Top with grilled apple slices.

apple cider vinaigrette
5 tablespoons sugar
¼ teaspoon dry mustard
5 tablespoons distilled white vinegar
3 teaspoons apple cider vinegar
1½ tablespoons Worcestershire sauce
3 tablespoons canola oil
Kosher salt and freshly ground black pepper
In a small plastic bowl, whisk together the sugar, dry mustard, white vinegar, apple cider vinegar, and then Worcestershire sauce until the sugar has dissolved. Slowly add the oil in a stream, whisking to emulsify—season with salt and pepper to taste.

Pear and spinach salad

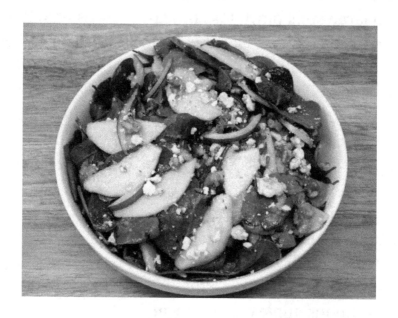

serves 4
ingredients.

¼ cup Basic Vinaigrette
2 p ears (preferably Bosc)
1 bag (6 ounces) Baby Spinach
¼ pound Gorgonzola, thinly sliced
¼ cup almond slices, toasted
Prepare the Basic Vinaigrette.

Description:

Peel the pears. Using a vegetable peeler, shave the pear meat into thin slivers.
Place the Baby Spinach in a large salad bowl.
Add vinaigrette and stir gently to coat. Divide the spinach among the plates.
Top with the pear shavings and Gorgonzola slices.
Sprinkle with the almonds.
Serve immediately.

Grapefruit and avocado salad

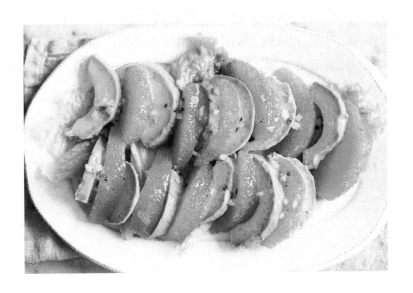

serves 4
ingredients:

1 grapefruit, peeled
½ white onion halved and thinly sliced
2 avocados peeled and cut
1 bag (7 ounces) Riviera™ Blend
3 tablespoons extra-virgin olive oil
Kosher salt and freshly ground pepper

Description:

Over a large plastic salad bowl, separate the grapefruit slices, catching the juice in the bowl. Remove the seeds. Add the grapefruit slices to the bowl. Add the onion, avocados, Riviera Blend, and olive oil and gently toss.
Season with salt and pepper to taste.

Waldorf salad

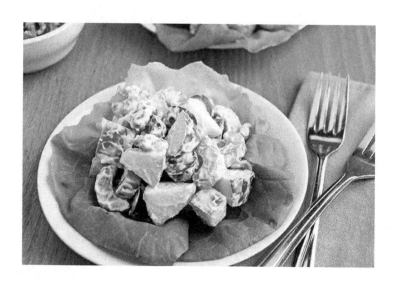

serves 4
ingredients:

2 Fuji apples, cored and cut in half
1 Red Delicious apple, cored and cut in half
3 tablespoons apple cider vinegar
¾ cup walnuts, toasted and coarsely chopped
1 cup raisins
2 teaspoons curry powder
2 celery stalks, thinly sliced
⅓ cup fresh mint, cut into thin strips
½ red onion halved and thinly sliced
1 cup mayonnaise

Kosher salt and freshly ground pepper
1 bag (10 ounces) Hearts of Romaine

Description:

Leaving the skin on for color, chop the apples into ¼-inch pieces.
In a large salad bowl, toss the apples with the cider vinegar.
Add the walnuts, raisins, curry powder, celery, mint, and red onion and toss. Fold in the mayonnaise to taste, to evenly coat. Season with salt and pepper to taste.
Cover and refrigerate until the flavors have melded, at least 1 hour.
To serve, arrange the Hearts of Romaine on individual plates and spoon the apple mixture on top.

Fresh fruit salad

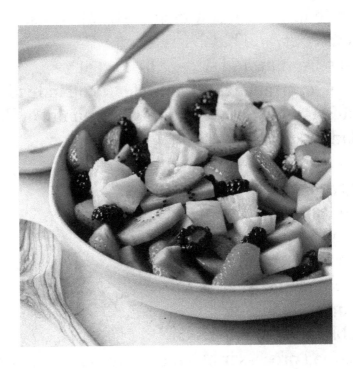

serves 4
ingredients:

½ cantaloupe, peeled, seeded, and diced
½ honeydew melon, peeled, seeded, and diced
½ cup fresh strawberries, hulled and thinly sliced
½ cup fresh raspberries
¼ cup fresh blueberries
1 bag (8 ounces) Triple Hearts™

Description:

In a large plastic salad bowl, gently toss together the
cantaloupe, honeydew melon, strawberries,
raspberries, and blueberries.
Add seasoning and stir gently to coat
To serve, arrange the Triple Hearts on individual
plates and top with a generous a spoonful of the fruit
salad.

poppy seed dressing
3 tablespoons red wine vinegar
⅓ cup sugar
1 teaspoon dry mustard
¾ teaspoon kosher salt
⅓ cup vegetable oil
1 tablespoon poppy seeds
In a food processor blend the vinegar, sugar, dry
mustard, salt and oil until well blended. Add the
poppy seeds.

Wildberry salad

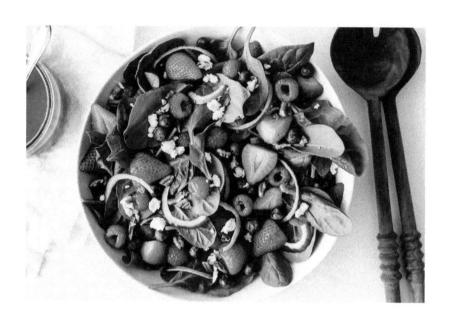

serves 4
ingredients:

1 bag (10 ounces) Baby Spinach
½ cup fresh blueberries
½ cup fresh raspberries
½ cup fresh blackberries
½ cup hulled and quartered fresh strawberries
Kosher salt and freshly ground pepper

Description:

In a large plastic salad bowl, toss together the Baby Spinach, blueberries, raspberries, blackberries, and strawberries.

Add the dressing to taste and gently toss—season with salt and pepper to taste. Serve immediately.

fresh raspberry dressing

½ cup fresh raspberries or frozen unsweetened raspberries

1 tablespoon apple juice

2 tablespoons raspberry balsamic vinegar

1¼ tablespoons water

1 tablespoon sugar

2 tablespoons canola oil

Kosher salt and freshly ground pepper

Place the raspberries, apple juice, vinegar, water, sugar, and oil in a blender.

Purée until smooth—season with salt and pepper to taste.

Tropical Fruit Salad

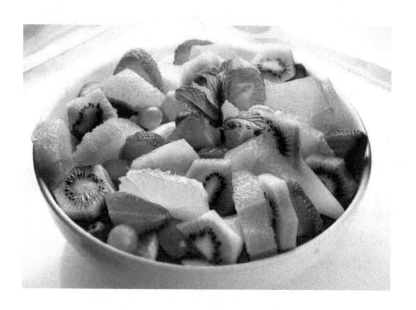

serves 4
ingredients:

1 bag (5 ounces) Baby Arugula
3 tablespoons coarsely chopped fresh mint leaves
1 mango, peeled, pitted, and sliced lengthwise
1 papaya, cut in half lengthwise, seeded, peeled, and sliced
lengthwise
8 pineapple slices (fresh or canned), cut in half

Description:

In a large plastic salad bowl, place the Baby Arugula
and mint leaves.
Add the dressing to taste and gently toss. Arrange the
slices of mango, papaya, and pineapple on individual
plates. Top with the salad.
Serve immediately.

passion fruit dressing

6 tablespoons medley of tropical fruit juice (must
include passion fruit juice)
1 tablespoon minced shallot
2 tablespoons extra-virgin olive oil
Kosher salt
In a small plastic bowl, whisk together the juice,
shallot, and oil until well combined.
Season with salt to taste.

CONCLUSIONS

Well, if you have come to this last page, it means that the salads have been to your liking and this makes me happy...

I am sure of one thing that I have not bored you with the usual recipes but believe me that I have put all possible effort to create salads that could surprise you but above all make you arrive at the goal...

Thank you for trusting me, and I send you an affectionate hug...

Eating Well to Feel Fit...

Robert Sorrento